YOUTH PHYSIOLOGY AND HYGIENE

M. B. Turopova, A. S. Bekmurodov

Youth Physiology and Hygiene

by: M. B. Turopova, A. S. Bekmurodov

Edition: December '2025

Publisher:

Taemeer Publications LLC (Michigan, USA / Hyderabad, India)

ISBN 978-93-6908-103-5

Book	:	Youth Physiology and Hygiene
Author	:	M. B. Turopova, A. S. Bekmurodov
Publisher	:	Taemeer Publications
Year	:	'2025
Pages	:	106
Title Design	:	*Taemeer Web Design*

Introduction

Today, major reforms are being implemented in the education system of our country. In particular, monitoring the health of the growing and developing young generation, determining the physical and mental capabilities of their bodies, studying the basics of their healthy lifestyle, radically changing the education system, and raising it to the level of modern requirements are among the urgent problems of today.

To provide modern knowledge, a teacher can first of all properly organize the educational process in educational institutions only when he understands the anatomical and physiological changes of the growing and developing generation at different times, as well as the hygienic significance of the impact of external environmental conditions on the child's body.

Students will gain the necessary experience in conducting practical classes in the field of youth physiology and hygiene, including hygienic assessment of students' physical development, study of spinal reflexes, reflex arc analysis, knee and Achilles reflexes, determination of active attention, speed of voluntary movement, mental performance, study of the effect of physical exertion on the activity of the cardiovascular and respiratory systems, k determination of visual acuity and visual field, to create a diet, Hygienic assessment of classrooms, workshops and gyms of educational institutions and their equipment, It is necessary to be able to practically apply the relevant scientific research methods in this subject in cases related to the hygiene of educational work, hygienic assessment of lessons and lesson schedules, hygienic assessment of the daily routine, and determination of the type of higher nervous activity. In this regard, this methodological guide serves to form students' knowledge and skills in the field of youth physiology and hygiene and to use them in their future activities.

Practical exercise 1. Hygienic assessment of the physical development of students

Purpose of the work: To study methods for checking anthropometric indicators in students and, based on the results obtained, to hygienically assess their physical development.

Educational equipment: Scales, height ruler, centimeter tape, spirometer, hand dynamometer.

Theoretical part: Anthropometric indicators are determined by conducting somotoscopic, somotometric, and physiometric examinations.

1. **Somotoscopy** (external observation) determines the elasticity of the skin, the development of skeletal muscles, and the normal development of the skeleton (chest, legs, stature). This examination takes into account the following:

a) The elasticity of the skin is determined by pulling the skin upwards with the thumb and index fingers and releasing it, that is, if no marks remain on the skin when the skin is released, the elasticity is considered good;

b) the development of the skeleton and muscles is determined visually, that is, if there are no deviations from the norm in the skeleton, and the shape of the muscles is noticeable (if they protrude from the skin), then it is considered developed;

c) the shape of the chest is observed visually, and cylindrical, conical, and flat shapes are determined;

g) The shape of the legs is determined by the contact of the knees and ankles, that is, if the thighs, calves, and knees touch each other, it is normal, if the ankles touch each other, it is an O-shaped leg, and if the knees touch, but the calves and ankles do not touch, it is an X-shaped leg;

d) Flat feet are determined by the shape of the footprint, that is, if the edges of the foot are flat and the middle part is not, it is normal, and if the entire part is flat, it is considered flat feet;

e) The shape of the body is visually observed, and the following body shapes are determined: normal, stooped (the head is slightly tilted forward, the shoulders hang forward, the chest is more concave, the belly protrudes forward), lordosis (the lumbar spine is bent forward more than normal, the belly protrudes), kyphosis (the shoulder blades are raised like wings, a hunched position), scoliosis (one shoulder is low, one is high).

2. **Somotometry** measures height (standing and sitting), weight, chest circumference, and head circumference.

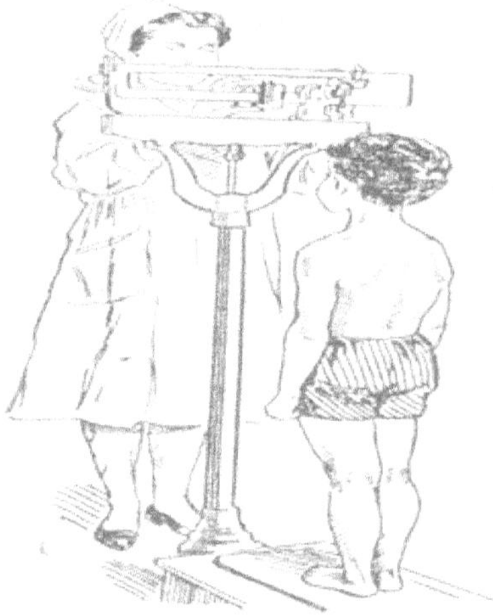

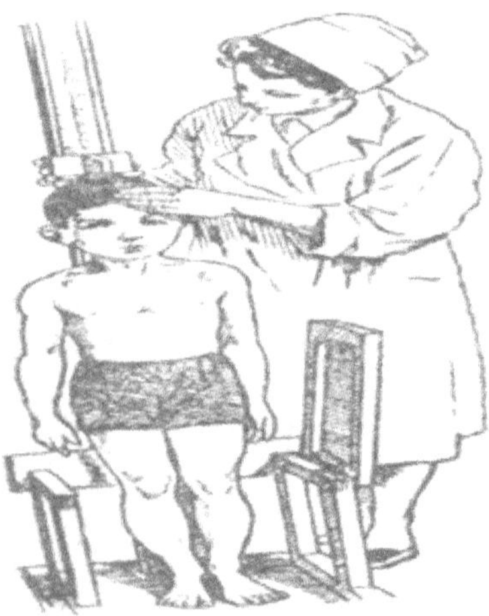

3. **Physiometry** determines physiological indicators. This examination method takes into account the following:

a) The vital capacity of the lungs is measured using a spirometer and compared with the following table:

Air type	Air volume (ml)
Breath to take air	500
Extra air	1500
Reserve air	1500
Lung vital capacity	3500

b) Muscle strength is measured using a hand dynamometer and compared with the table below.

Age	Right hand		Left hand	
	Son	**Girl**	**Son**	**Girl**
6	9.2	8.4	8.5	7.7

7	10.7	9.9	10.1	9.2
8	13.4	11.2	11.7	10.5
9	14.3	13.8	13.5	12
10	16.5	14.6	15.6	13.7
11	18.8	16.5	17.7	15.5
12	21.2	18.9	19.7	17.8
13	24.4	21.8	22.5	20.4
14	28.4	24.8	25.2	22.9
15	33.4	27	30.9	24.9
Adults	49.3	29.7	45	37.7

Control questions:

1. How are skin elasticity, skeletal muscle development, and normal skeleton development determined?

2. What instrument is used to measure the vital capacity of the lungs?

3. What instrument is used to measure muscle strength?

Practical exercise 2. Study of spinal reflexes. Analysis of the reflex arc, knee and Achilles reflexes

Objective: To study the effects of spinal reflexes and physical exertion on the cardiovascular system through experiments.

Training equipment: Hanging stand, tools for preparing the preparation, stopwatch, cotton, hook, 0.5 and 1% solutions of hydrochloric acid, 1% novocaine, water, saline, live frog.

Theoretical part: *Determining spinal reflexes.*

1. The frog is cut off only its brain and hung from the lower jaw on a tripod. Pour 0.5% hydrochloric acid into a small beaker and immerse the frog's hind leg in this solution. At this time, it withdraws its leg, then the skin of the calf is cut off in the form of a ring and peeled off. After 1-2 minutes, the same leg of the frog is

exposed to 0.5% hydrochloric acid again. But this time it cannot withdraw its leg, because now the receptor, that is, one element of the reflex arc, has been removed. If the leg whose skin has not been cut, is exposed to a stronger solution of acid, not only this leg, but also the other leg and the whole body of the frog will move.

2. After seeing that the frog has a reflex in its spinal cord, the skin on the back of the thigh of one of its legs is cut and the sciatic nerve is found between the muscles. A thread is passed under it. Then, even if this leg is immersed in a strong solution of acid, it does not contract, that is, the reflex is not formed due to the destruction of the efferent nerve fiber. This can also be observed by exposing this nerve to novocaine, in which the sciatic nerve loses its sensitivity under the influence of novocaine in 1-2 minutes.

3. A special wire is inserted into the spinal canal to disrupt the nervous system. After that,

even if the frog's leg is exposed to acid, it will not have a reflex.

Observing proprioceptive reflexes in humans

Reflexes that occur as a result of the action of receptors located in muscles, tendons, and joints in humans are called proprioceptive reflexes. These include the knee reflex and the Achilles tendon reflex.

1. **Knee reflex.** The person being examined sits with his legs crossed. If the tendon of his quadriceps muscle is gently tapped with a special hammer, the calf muscles (leg) are recorded. In this case, the reflex arc is located around the III-IV lumbar segments.

2. **Achilles** To test **the reflex** , the person being examined sits on a chair with their knees bent. If the Achilles tendon is gently tapped with a hammer, the toes are flexed, with the reflex arc extending around the I-II calcaneal segments.

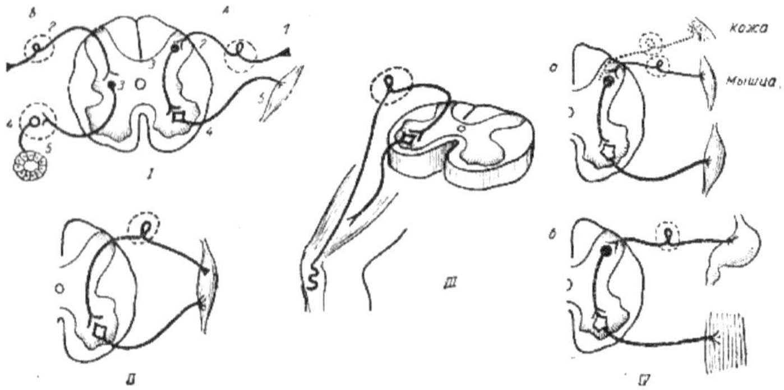

Control questions:

1. Distinguish between unconditioned and conditioned reflexes.

2. What is seen as the reflex arc in the knee reflex?

3. What is seen as the reflex arc in the Achilles reflex?

4. Sensory nerve cell, motor nerve cell spinal cord

In which branches is it located?

Tasks:

1. Write down the processes by which a frog responds to stimuli.

Head brain broken				Back brain broken
If 0.5% hydrochloric acid is applied to the hind leg	Baldir skin ring in the form of sly taken leg to acid if touched	Skin uncut on the leg acid stronger solution with impact if possible	If a frog's leg is exposed to acid by severing its nerve,	Frog leg to acid if touched

2. Conduct an experiment to observe proprioceptive reflexes in humans and write down the results.

3rd practical training. Determining active attention, speed of voluntary movement, and mental performance

Purpose of the work: To consolidate students' knowledge about active attention, voluntary movement speed, and mental performance through experiments and testing.

Educational equipment: 4 random number tables (10x10) from 1 to 25, stopwatch, correction chart.

Theoretical part: ***Determining the speed of voluntary movement***

The level of development of the child's nervous and muscular systems is determined by the speed of voluntary movements of the hand and paw. To do this, each student draws three 10x10 rectangles on a white sheet of paper.

When the command "Let's start" is given,

each student must place as many dots as possible and as quickly as possible inside the first rectangle. After 10 seconds, the command "stop" is given and the work is stopped. This experiment is repeated three times. Then each student counts the dots inside the rectangle and writes them down next to it, which is the average result. To do this, the results are added up and divided by the number of experiments. The average result is compared with the table.

Age		7	8	9	10	11	12	13	14	15	16	17	18
Number of points	Son	40	45	52	56	58	60	63	65	67	70	75	80
	Girl	35	38	41	44	47	51	53	55	55	62	66	72

The following formula is used to calculate the percentage of work done.

$$\frac{A \times 100\%}{C}$$

Where: A is the student's average score;

C is the overall average for age (table).

A student's average score that differs from the overall score by ±15% indicates that the speed of voluntary movement is within normal limits.

Identifying active attention

The concentration and duration of active attention depend on the age of adolescents. The younger the child, the slower the inhibition process and the faster the excitation is radiated in the cerebral hemispheres. The duration of active attention is 15 minutes at 7-8 years old, 20 minutes at 9-10 years old, 25 minutes at 11-12 years old, 30 minutes at 13-14 years old, 40 minutes at 15-16 years old, and around 55-60 minutes in adults. If mental work lasts longer than necessary, the student becomes restless, and the accuracy and speed of mental work decreases. Therefore, it is necessary to change the type of mental work several times during the lesson. The more concentrated the active attention, the faster and more accurately the mental work is performed.

The concentration of active attention can be determined by the speed of finding the numbers presented in the table (1,2,3,4– table).

Table 1

1	15	6	13	8
10	21	23	18	4
19	24	2	25	20
12	7	22	11	16
3	14	17	5	9

Table 2

13	15	5	7	1
2	20	23	21	9
18	6	11	25	17
22	24	19	12	3
16	4	8	14	10

3 – table

12	4	25	23	14
15	21	8	10	5
6	19	1	13	16
17	11	24	22	2
3	9	20	7	18

Table 4

1	7	11	14	16
13	21	19	25	2
20	15	8	5	10
3	18	24	17	22
23	9	4	12	6

Each of the examiners is given tables 1,2,3,4 and instructed to find (erase) the numbers from 1 to 25 in order. They are told to find the numbers as quickly as possible. The examiner starts the numbers in table 1 by running a stopwatch and the time it takes to find (erase) the numbers is determined. The same experiment is conducted with tables 2,3,4 and the average is determined. To calculate the average, the times from 4 tables are added and divided by 4. For example, 120 seconds were spent on 4 tables, 120 : 4 = 30.

If the numbers 1 to 25 written on the table can be found in 30-40 seconds, the concentration of attention is considered good, if it is found in 45-60 seconds, it is satisfactory, and finally, if it is found in more than 60 seconds, it is considered unsatisfactory.

Determining a person's mental performance during activities that require attention

Currently, a correction table (Anfimov table) is widely used to determine the IQ. Working with this table requires accuracy, speed, and concentration.

During the experiment, both qualitative and quantitative aspects of the work are evaluated. The results of the experiment are determined using the following formulas.

A = A- accuracy coefficient;

M - the number of deleted letters;

H – number of letters seen.

P =A× C P – AIQ coefficient;

C is the total number of letters seen.

Students are given the Anfimov table. They

must mark 1 letter in the table for 4 minutes. This experiment is repeated with all the letters in the table. Speed, attention, and accuracy are required during the work. The marked letters are counted separately and the following table is filled in.

Working hours	Given letters	Number of letters found in 4 minutes	Available in the table number of letters	Total and found difference in the number of letters

Speed is judged by the total number of symbols considered in 4 minutes, and accuracy is judged by the total number of errors made in 4 minutes.

Anfimov schedule

C	X	A	B	C	X	E	B	I	X	H	A	I	C	H	X	B	K	C	H	A	I	C	B	X	B	E	H	A	I	C	K	E	B	I
X	H	B	C	H	A	B	C	A	B	C	H	A	E	K	E	A	X	B	K	E	C	B	C	H	A	I	C	A	I	C	H	A	I	H
X	I	C	X	B	X	E	K	B	X	I	B	X	E	I	C	I	E	I	H	A	I	E	H	K	X	K	I	K	X	E	K	B	K	I
C	X	A	K	X	H	C	K	A	I	C	B	E	K	B	X	H	A	I	C	H	X	E	K	A	I	C	H	A	K	C	K	B	X	B
K	X	B	H	A	I	C	I	X	A	E	X	C	X	B	X	E	K	B	X	I	B	X	E	I	C	I	E	I	H	A	I	E	H	K
X	K	I	K	X	E	K	B	K	I	C	X	A	K	X	H	C	K	A	I	C	B	E	K	B	X	H	A	I	C	H	X	E	K	A
I	C	H	A	K	C	K	B	X	B	K	X	B	H	A	I	C	I	X	A	E	X	H	A	E	K	E	A	X	B	K	E	C	B	C
H	A	I	C	A	I	C	H	A	I	H	X	I	C	X	B	X	E	K	B	X	I	B	X	E	I	X	B	E	H	A	I	C	K	E
B	I	X	H	B	C	H	A	B	C	A	B	C	H	A	E	K	E	A	X	B	K	E	C	B	C	H	A	I	C	A	I	C	H	A
I	H	X	I	C	X	B	X	E	K	B	X	I	B	X	E	I	C	I	E	I	H	A	I	E	H	K	X	K	I	K	X	E	K	B
K	I	C	X	A	K	X	H	C	K	A	I	C	B	E	K	B	X	H	A	I	C	H	B	H	A	I	C	I	X	A	E	X	H	A
E	K	E	A	X	B	K	E	C	B	C	H	A	I	C	A	I	C	H	A	I	H	X	I	C	X	B	X	E	K	B	X	I	B	X
E	I	X	B	E	H	A	I	C	K	E	B	I	X	H	B	C	H	A	B	C	A	B	E	X	C	X	B	X	E	K	B	X	I	B
X	E	I	C	I	E	I	H	A	I	E	H	K	X	K	I	K	X	E	K	B	K	I	C	X	A	K	X	H	C	K	A	I	C	B
E	K	B	X	H	A	I	C	H	X	E	K	A	I	C	H	A	K	C	K	B	X	B	K	X	B	H	A	I	C	I	X	A	E	X
H	A	E	K	E	A	X	B	K	E	C	B	C	H	A	I	C	A	I	C	H	A	I	H	X	I	C	X	B	X	E	K	B	X	I
B	X	E	I	X	B	E	H	A	I	C	K	E	B	I	X	H	B	C	H	A	B	C	A	B	C	H	A	E	K	E	A	X	B	K
C	B	C	H	A	I	C	A	I	C	H	A	I	H	X	I	C	X	B	X	E	K	B	X	I	B	X	E	I	C	I	E	I	H	A
I	E	H	K	X	K	I	K	X	E	K	B	K	I	C	X	A	K	X	H	C	K	A	I	C	B	E	K	B	X	H	A	I	C	H
B	H	A	I	C	I	X	A	E	X	H	A	E	K	E	A	X	B	K	E	C	B	C	H	A	I	C	A	I	C	H	A	I	H	X
I	C	X	B	X	E	K	B	X	I	B	X	E	I	X	B	E	H	A	I	C	I	X	A	E	X	C	X	B	X	E	K	B	X	I
B	X	E	I	C	I	E	I	H	A	I	E	H	K	X	K	I	K	X	E	K	B	K	I	C	X	A	K	X	H	C	K	A	I	C
B	E	K	B	X	H	A	I	C	H	X	E	K	A	I	C	H	A	K	C	K	B	X	B	K	X	B	H	A	I	C	I	X	A	E
X	H	A	E	K	E	A	X	B	K	E	C	B	C	H	A	I	A	B	C	X	E	B	I	X	H	A	I	C	H	X	B	K	C	H
A	I	C	B	X	B	E	H	A	I	C	K	E	B	I	X	H	B	C	H	K	B	K	I	C	X	A	K	X	H	C	K	A	I	C
B	E	K	B	X	H	A	I	C	H	X	E	K	A	I	C	H	A	K	C	K	B	X	B	K	X	B	H	A	I	C	I	X	A	E
X	H	A	E	K	E	A	X	B	K	E	C	B	C	H	A	I	A	B	C	X	E	B	I	X	H	A	I	C	H	X	B	K	C	H
A	C	C	B	X	B	C	H	A	I	C	I	E	B	I	X	H	B	X	B	K	X	B	H	A	I	C	I	X	A	E	X	H	A	I
K	E	A	X	B	K	E	C	B	C	H	A	I	A	B	C	X	E	B	I	X	H	A	I	C	H	X	B	K	C	H	A	I	C	B
X	B	E	H	A	I	C	K	E	B	I	X	H	B	C	H	K	K	E	A	X	B	K	E	C	B	C	H	A	I	C	A	I	C	H
A	I	H	X	I	C	X	B	X	E	K	B	X	I	B	X	E	I	C	I	E	I	H	A	I	E	H	K	X	K	I	K	X	E	K
B	K	I	C	X	A	K	X	H	C	K	A	I	C	B	E	K	B	X	H	A	I	C	H	B	H	A	I	C	I	X	A	E	X	H
A	E	K	E	A	X	B	K	E	C	B	C	H	A	I	C	A	I	C	H	A	I	H	X	I	C	X	B	X	E	K	B	A	I	B
X	E	I	X	B	E	H	A	I	C	I	X	A	E	X	C	X	B	X	E	K	B	X	I	B	X	E	I	C	I	E	I	H	A	I
E	H	K	X	K	I	K	X	E	K	B	K	I	C	X	C	X	B	X	E	K	B	X	I	B	X	E	I	C	I	E	I	H	A	I
H	K	X	K	I	K	X	E	K	B	K	I	C	X	A	K	X	H	C	K	A	I	C	B	E	K	B	X	H	A	I	C	H	B	H
A	I	C	I	X	A	E	X	H	A	E	K	E	A	X	B	K	E	C	B	C	H	A	I	C	A	I	C	H	A	I	H	X	I	C
X	B	X	E	K	B	X	I	B	X	E	I	X	B	E	H	A	I	C	K	E	B	I	X	H	B	C	H	A	B	C	A	B	E	X
C	X	D	X	E	K	B	Y	I	B	X	E	I	C	I	E	I	H	A	I	E	H	K	X	K	I	K	X	C	K	A	I	C	B	E

Tasks:

1. With the teacher's command, place dots inside the squares, determine the average, and calculate the percentage of voluntary movement based on the table.

$$\frac{A \times 100\%}{C}$$

A – the student's average result; C– overall average (table)

<table>
<tr><td>

</td><td>

</td></tr>
<tr><td>Number of points No. 1 ________</td><td>Number of points No. 2 ________</td></tr>
<tr><td>

</td><td>

</td></tr>
<tr><td>Number of points No. 3 ________</td><td>Number of points No. 4 ________</td></tr>
<tr><td colspan="2">Average __________________ Percentage indicator ________</td></tr>
</table>

2. Find the numbers in the tables in sequence, determine the time, and find the average.

Table 1

1	15	6	13	8
10	21	23	18	4
19	24	2	25	20
12	7	22	11	16
3	14	17	5	9

Table 2

13	15	5	7	1
2	20	23	21	9
18	6	11	25	17
22	24	19	12	3
16	4	8	14	10

3 – table

12	4	25	23	14
15	21	8	10	5
6	19	1	13	16
17	11	24	22	2
3	9	20	7	18

Table 4

1	7	11	14	16
13	21	19	25	2
20	15	8	5	10
3	18	24	17	22
23	9	4	12	6

Your average is _____ Group average is ____

3. Work with the Anfimov table and fill in the table based on the results obtained.

Working hours	Given letters	Number of letters found in 4 minutes	Available in the table number of letters	Total and found difference in letter numbers
	A		160	
	B		176	
	E		146	
	I		202	
	K		153	
	N		144	
	S		175	
	X		209	

4. The results of the experiment are determined using the following formulas.

A =

A- accuracy coefficient;

M - the number of deleted

letters;

H – number of letters seen.

P – AIQ coefficient;

$P = A \times C$

C is the total number of letters seen.

4th practical exercise. Studying the effects of physical activity on the cardiovascular and respiratory systems

Purpose of the work: to study the effect of physical activity on the cardiovascular and respiratory systems.

Educational equipment: stopwatch, blood pressure monitor, phonendoscope, spirometer.

Theoretical part: ***Studying the effects of physical activity on the heart and vascular system***

The most pronounced pulse is determined by placing 4 fingers of the right hand on the area of the carpal artery of the subject. After that, the pulse - the number of heartbeats - is determined for one minute. The number of arterial pulse beats per minute is determined three times and the average is calculated (the average number of pulses in a healthy person is 72-85 per minute).

After the subject has sat up for the 10th time, the pulse is counted again. The results at rest and after physical exertion are compared.

Lung vital capacity

When a person breathes calmly, he inhales and exhales from 500/300 to 900 ml of air. This air is called tidal air. After a normal breath, an additional 1500 ml of air can be inhaled, which is called supplementary air. After a normal exhalation, another 1500 ml of air can be exhaled. This is called the reserve part of the exhalation. The vital capacity of the lungs is the maximum volume of air exhaled after a deep breath. Normally, the vital capacity of the lungs is 2700 ml in women and 3500 ml in men. Even after a maximum exhalation, some air remains in the lungs. This is called residual air and is around 1200 ml.

Spirometry is a method of measuring the vital capacity of the lungs. The spirometer device consists of 2 cylinders. The outer cylinder is filled with water to the mark, and the second is empty, with an air-filled balloon attached to its base. A metal tube is passed through the outer cylinder, through which the subject breathes. Light breathing is also transmitted to the balloon, raising the inner cylinder. The counting symbol is shown separately.

The spirometer is set to “0”. The mouthpiece at the end of the metal tube is rinsed in a manganese solution. The subject stands in front of the spirometer, takes a deep breath 2-3 times, exhales, takes another deep breath and exhales into the spirometer (as hard as possible). The breath should be continuous and slow.

Determination of additional air . A probe is removed from the cylinder cap, and the inner cylinder is manually raised to the 3000 ml mark. After taking several calm breaths, the subject pauses for a moment, places the mouthpiece in his mouth and takes a deep breath into the spirometer. The inner cylinder how many up to the mark down fallen is determined and take from 3000 is thrown away . additional air become is considered .

Breath the air to determine . Spirometer set to "0" is brought . The one being examined mouthpiece into the mouth take it , calm down in case the air nose through take a breath to the spirometer It does this 5-6 times. returned , received of numbers average is determined .

Reserve the air Set the spirometer to "0" position . is brought . Several times quiet breath from receiving then breath take out a little from stopping then mouthpiece into the mouth can take until harder breath to the spirometer The number on the scale is the reserve . air size shows . The work at the end additional , reserve and breath the weather adding , previous determined vitality capacity amount with are compared . Results the difference does not exceed 10% need .

Control questions:

1. What do you understand by vital capacity of the lungs?
2. What instrument is used to measure the vital capacity of the lungs?
3. What is the normal vital capacity of the lungs in women?
4. What is the normal vital capacity of the lungs in men?
5. What does the lung's vital capacity depend on?

Tasks:

1. Count your arterial pulse in 1 minute and fill in the table.

1 minute arterial pulses number (normal 72–85 t a)					Physical from scratch after	
1st time	2nd time	3 times	Average	Group average	Personal	Group average

2. Spirometer using of the lungs vitality capacity measure the table fill in and to the norm compare .

Air type	Air volume (ml)	
	Result	Norm (average)
Breath to take air		500
Extra air		1500

Reserve air		1500
Lung vital capacity		3500

Practical exercise 5. Determining visual acuity and visual field

Objective: To study the technique of determining visual acuity using the Golovin table and the visual field using a perimeter instrument.

Educational equipment: Golovin table, meter, indicator, perimeter, reflection of the projection of hemispheres, pencil, colored markers, ruler, paper.

Theoretical part: Visual acuity is the ability of the eye to see two points of light separately. A normal eye is able to see two points of light separately at an angle of 1°. Seeing two points separately is associated with the fact that at least one pupil is excited between two excited pupils. The diameter of the pupil is 3 μm, and in order to see two points separately, the image of these two points should be no less than 4 μm in the quadrature, and then the image size will be when the viewing angle is 1°. Therefore, if two points of light are seen when the viewing angle is less than 1°, the points will merge.

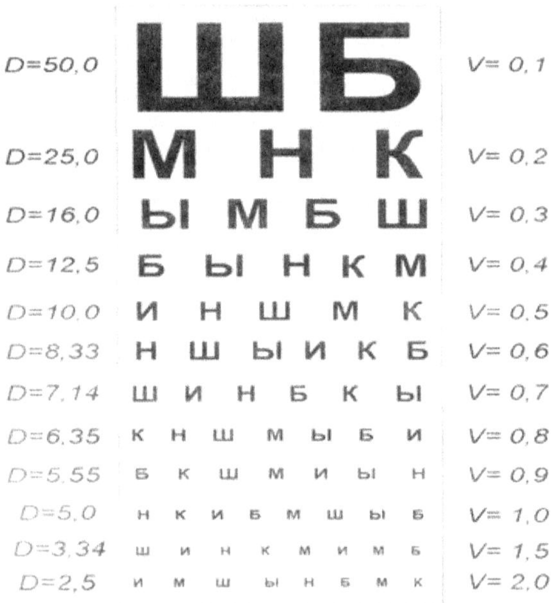

D=50,0 Ш Б V= 0,1
D=25,0 М Н К V= 0,2
D=16,0 Ы М Б Ш V= 0,3
D=12,5 Б Ы Н К М V= 0,4
D=10,0 И Н Ш М К V= 0,5
D=8,33 Н Ш Ы И К Б V= 0,6
D=7,14 Ш И Н Б К Ы V= 0,7
D=6,35 К Н Ш М Ы Б И V= 0,8
D=5,55 Б К Ш М И Ы Н V= 0,9
D=5,0 Н К И Б М Ш Ы Б V= 1,0
D=3,34 Ш И Н К М И М Б V= 1,5
D=2,5 И М Ш Ы Н Б М К V= 2,0

Golovin's schedule

To determine visual acuity, a standard table (Golovin table) consisting of 12 rows of letter symbols is used. The size of the letters decreases from top to bottom. The number next to each row indicates the distance at which a normal eye should see the letters in this row separately when the visual angle is 1°. The table is hung on a well-lit wall (illumination should not be less than 10 lux) or illuminated by an additional electric lamp. The subject is seated on a chair 5 meters from the table and is offered to cover one eye with a special device (shit). The examiner shows the letters on a stick to the examinee and asks him to name them. The determination begins with the top row, the lowest row is found, and the examinee is asked to see the letters clearly and clearly for 2-3 s and name them. The row in which there is an error is ignored, and the row one above it is considered. Then, the visual acuity (visus) is calculated based on the following formula:

$$V = \frac{a}{D};$$

In this: V - visual acuity, a - the distance between the examinee and the table, D - The distance at which a normal eye must clearly see the letters in this row.

After that, the visual acuity of the other eye is determined.

Determining the field of view

When the eye is focused on a point, the surrounding area visible to the eye is called the visual field. The visual field varies in people, depending on the shape of the eye, the depth of its location, the shape of the eyebrows and nose, and the functional state of the retina. There is a distinction between the color (chromatic) and colorless (achromatic) visual fields. Achromatic vision is larger than the chromatic visual field, since achromatic vision is associated with the activity of the rods located mainly in the periphery of the retina. The visual field is not the same for different colors, but is largest for yellow and narrowest for green.

The boundaries of the achromatic field of view are as follows: from the outside - up to 100°, from the inside and above - 60°, and from the bottom - 65°.

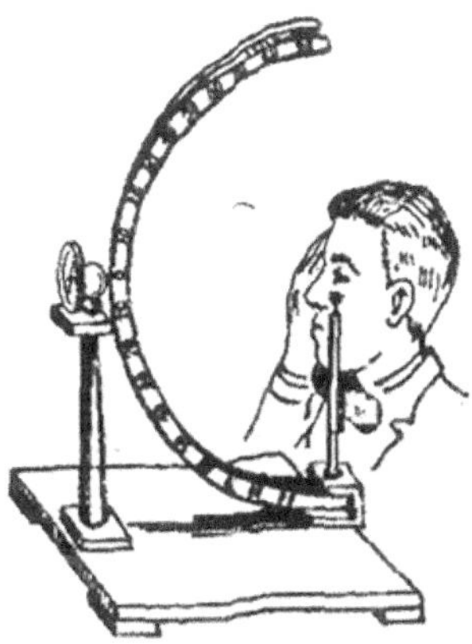

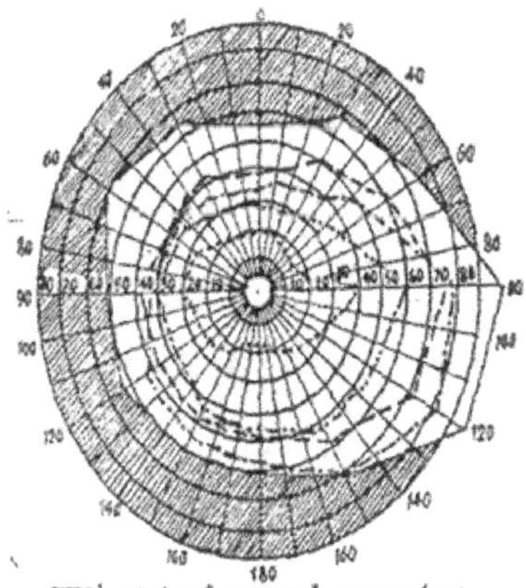

Achromatic and chromatic see of the area penmetric photo . Conditional characters : 1) black and white see area ; 2) for yellow color see area ; 3) for blue see area ; 4) for red color see area ; 5) for green see area .

View area *Forster perimeter* using is determined . Perimeter light opposite is installed . Checked to the light relatively back side with after sitting , perimeter tripod carved to the place chin If the left eye see area identifiable if yes , chin base (podstavka) right to the part is placed . The base height so is managed , in which eye of the cup bottom border tripod high to the border correct comes . The one being checked gaze perimeter in the center white to the point directed without , second eye hand with closure need .

Perimeter arc horizontal to the situation placed , measured begins . This for white stamp of the arc internal surface from 90° to 0° along side slowly take bride and under investigation white to the point looking at standing without the stamp seeing to say needed . Checker correct arrived the corner define , second times again examines . Eye how much many meridian according to see area If it is clear , it is clear. will be .

This method occupying to take There are 2 main meridians for : horizontal (external , internal) and vertically (top , bottom) determination with limitation possible .

White stamp colored to thc stamp replaced , above to the method mainly color vision area is determined and under investigation only the stamp without seeing , maybe his/her the color is also clear knowledge need . View the area blue or one how many in colors determination possible .

View of the area boundaries :

Direction	View of the area white to color	In degrees size green to color
From above		
From below		
From outside		
From the inside		

Received to the results based on 2 color for see the area draw , white and green colors for see the area compare and they between differences the reason Explain .

Control questions:

1. What is visual acuity?

2. What is the field of view?

3. How is achromatic vision different from chromatic vision?

4. What instrument is used to determine the field of view?

Tasks:

1. Record the data obtained based on the Golovin table.

Eye	Distance between table and examinee	Viewed row	Distance written next to the line	Visual acuity
Right eye				
Left eye				

1. Fill in the table and graph it based on the information obtained based on the perimeter.

Eye	White plate	Yellow plate	Green colored plate

	Towards the nose	Outer side	High	Low	Towards the nose	Outer side	High	Low	Towards the nose	Outer side	High	Low
Right eye												
Left eye												

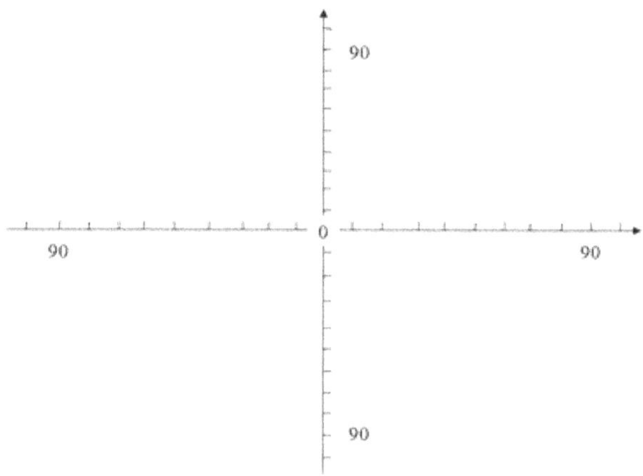

right eye

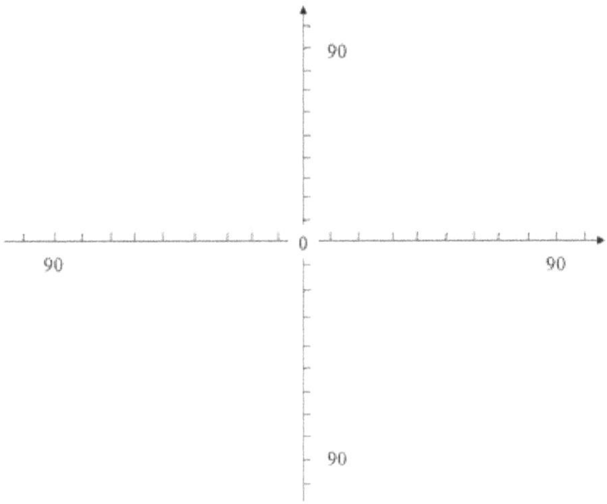

left eye

Practical exercise 6. Creating a diet

Objective: To develop students' skills in planning their diet based on their daily energy expenditure.

Teaching aids: A table showing the chemical composition of foods and how many calories they contain.

Theoretical part: Four meals a day is the

best diet. It is advisable that the first, morning breakfast should account for 25-30% of the total calories, lunch for 35-40%, second lunch for 10-15%, and dinner for 15-20%. It is advisable to eat protein-rich foods (meat, fish, eggs) for breakfast and lunch. For dinner, dairy and green products should be left. At least 50% of the proteins and fats entering the body should be from animal products. At the same time, the diet should include a sufficient amount of vitamins, mineral salts and water.

A diet is created using a table that shows the percentage of proteins, fats, and carbohydrates in a food and how many calories are in 100 g of food. If the amount of proteins, fats, and carbohydrates in the daily diet does not meet the norm, then the nutrients should be increased or decreased accordingly.

Distribution of daily food calorie intake by meal (in %)

Mealtime	Younger students	Older students
Breakfast	20-25	25-30
Lunch	30-35	3 5 -40
Second lunch	20	10-15
Dinner	20-25	15 -2 0

To the profession looking at expendable energy amount determination for people into 4 groups is divided .

First group – few physical power spenders – scientists , engineers , administrators employees , tailors , mechanics , students , teachers , doctors . Daily energy Consumption 2500-2800 kcal .

Second group – turners , weavers , mail employees , laboratory employees . Daily energy Consumption 3000 kcal .

The third group - those who spend a lot of physical effort - blacksmiths, carpenters, fitters, workers. Daily energy expenditure is 3500-4000 kcal.

The fourth group - those who perform heavy physical labor - porters, foresters, diggers, miners. Daily energy expenditure is 4500-5000 kcal.

The amount of protein, fat, carbohydrates, and energy in various foods

No.	Food products	Amount of protein, fat, and carbohydrates in 100 g of food product (g)			100 g of food in the product energy amount (
		protein	oil	carbohydrates	
1	Beef	20.2	7.0 g	—	187
2	Chicken meat	17.2	12.3	—	185
3	Fish	16.0	0.7	—	72
4	Egg (1 piece)	12.5	12.1	0.55	175
5	Milk	2.8	3.5	4.5	65
6	Yogurt	2.8	3.5	2.9	56
7	Cottage cheese	11.1	18.9	2.3	230
8	Cheese	22.6	25.7	—	332
9	White bread	6.7	0.7	50.3	240
10	Black bread	5.3	1.2	46.1	222

11	Rice	6.4	0.9	72.5	332
12	Pasta	9.3	0.8	70.9	336
13	Peas	19.8	2.2	50.8	310
14	Beans	19.6	2.0	51.4	310
15	Sugar	—	—	95.5	390
16	Potato	2.4	0.22	19.5	62.5
17	Carrot	1.2	0.3	9.0	30.5
18	Tomato	0.5	—	4.0	18
19	Cucumber	0.7	—	2.9	15
20	Apple	0.3	—	10.8	45

Daily food intake

Products name	Children's age					
	6 months 1 year old	1-3 young	3 -7 young	7- 11 young	11 - 15 young	15-18 young
Black bread	-	10	50	50	100	135
White wheat bread	12.5	40	100	150	250	315
Pasta product	-	5	5	10	20	10
Potato	50	100	200	250	325	325
Vegetables	100	140	200	275	325	325
Fresh fruits	160	200	200	250	250	250
Dried fruits	-	10	20	20	20	20
Sugar	45	50	60	60	80	100
Sweets	-	10	10	15	20	20
Vegetable oil , margarine	-	-	2	5	5	10
Tea	-	0.1	0.3	0.3	0.3	0.8
Cocoa	-	0.5	1	1.0	1	0.5
Coffee	–	1	3	3	3	3.5
Meat products	10	60	80	180	120	200

Fish product	-	-	40	50	50	50
Milk	500	600	500	500	500	500
Butter	5	20	23	35	30	25
Cottage cheese	15	30	30	35	25	30
Sour cream	-	10	15	15	15	20
Cheese	-	5	10	10	10	20
Egg (yolk)	4	25	50	50	50	50

The norm of protein, fat, and carbohydrates in a daily diet for children and adolescents

Children and teenagers age	Food substances quantity (g)			Energy released from these substances
	protein	oil	carbohydrates	
1-1.5 years old	44-55	44-45	160-175	1300
1.5-3	52-55	32-55	225	1600
3-5	58-60	58 -60	260	18-10
5-7	65-75	75-80	250-300	1800-2300
8-11	75-90	80-90	350-400	2400-2800
12-14	90-100	90-100	400-450	2800-3200
16-18	100-120	100-110	450-500	3200-3500
Big people	100-120	80-110	450-500	3200-3500

The amount of vitamins the body needs per day

	Vitamins (mg) (on account of h)					
	A	B_1	B	C	RR	*D*

			2			
Big old man	1	1-3	2	30-75	12-20	Up to 0.04
Pregnant, lactating women	2-2.5	3	2	75-100	18-20	0.16-0.32
7 years old was children	1	1	2	33	12	0.16-0.32
7 years old big children	1	1.5-2	2	50	12	0.16-0.32

Age groups	B_1	B_2	RR	B_6	C	A	D
	mg					mg	mg
0.5-1 year	0.5	0.6	0.6	0.5	20	0.5	
1 -1.5 years old	0.8	1.1	9 .0	1 .9	35	1.0	
1-2.5 years	0.9	1.2	10.0	1.0	40	1.0	
3-4 years old	1.1	1.4	12.0	1.3	45	1.0	
5-6 young	1.2	1.6	13.0	1.4	50	1.0	
7-10 years old	1.4	1.9	15.0	1.7	50	1.5	0.16
11 - 13 years old	1.7	2.3	19.0	2.0	60	1.5	
14-17 years old (teenagers)	1.0	2.5	21.0	2.2	80	1.5	
14-17 years old (girls)	1.7	2.2	18.0	1.9	70	1.5	

Control questions:

1. Explain the exchange of matter and energy.
2. What are the main food ingredients?

3. What should you pay attention to when creating a diet?

4. What is the daily protein requirement?

5. How much fat do you need per day?

Tasks:

1. Create a breakfast diet (average 960 kcal)

No.	Product type	Weight (grams)	Protein	Oil	Carbohydrate	Calories (kcal)
			in grams			
1						
2						
3						
4						
5						
6						

2. Lunch diet make (average 1280 kcal)

No.	Product type	Weight (grams)	Protein	Oil	Carbohydrate	Calories (kcal)
			in grams			

1						
2						
3						
4						
5						
6						
7						
8						

3. Create a second lunch menu (average 320 kcal)

No.	Product type	Weight (grams)	Protein	Oil	Carbohydrate	Calories (kcal)
			in grams			
1						
2						
3						
4						

4. Create a dinner menu (average 640 kcal)

No.	Product type	Weight (grams)	Protein	Oil	Carbohydrate	Calories (kcal)
			in grams			
1						

2						
3						
4						
5						
6						

7 th practical exercise. Hygienic assessment of classrooms, workshops and gyms of educational institutions and their equipment

Purpose of the work: to collect information about the equipment and dimensions of classrooms, workshops, and gyms, and to conduct a hygienic assessment based on standards.

Educational equipment: meter, centimeter tape, tables reflecting the norm.

Theoretical part: If the desk is adjusted to the student's height, it will be convenient to perform writing, reading, and drawing exercises, and the student's body, chest, and spine will develop normally. On the contrary, when the student performs exercises at a desk that is not adjusted to his height, he will feel discomfort, get tired quickly, and his handwriting will be impaired. Finally, as a result of sitting at such a desk for several months or years, the spine and chest will become curved, and the student's physique will be distorted.

The student is required to sit at a desk or table that is appropriate for their height, with their body upright and their head slightly tilted forward, with the distance between their eyes and the notebook or book being 35-40 cm, their back touching (leaning) against the back of the desk or chair, with a space between their chest and the edge of the desk cover that can accommodate the palm of their hand, and with the soles of their feet comfortably touching the floor.

School equipment includes: desk, table, chair, blackboard. The distance between the eyes and the table should be 35-40 cm. The slope of the desk should be 12-150. The front desks should be placed at least 2.5 meters from the wall and blackboard. Desks and tables should be light gray, light yellow, white and black colors are not recommended. Until 1971, desks were produced in 7 numbers according to the state standard (GOST). When producing them, the height of children was differentiated every 10 cm, that is, from 110 cm to 179 cm, desks were from number 6 to number 12.

Currently, five groups (A, B, C, D) of desks, tables, and chairs are produced. This group is determined by the following formula:

$$\text{№} = \frac{\text{бўй} - 100}{15}$$

in this – height – of the child tall

№– desk number

15– the inclination of the table .

Desks, table groups and sizes

Child's height (cm)	Desk, table and table group	Color marking	Desk cover height	Desk chair height of
130	A (1)	Yellow	54	32
130–145	B (2)	Red	60	36
145–160	B (3)	Light blue	66	40
160–175	G (4)	Green	72	44
175	D (5)	White	78	48

The classroom blackboard depends on the grade level and should be from 175 cm to 300-350 cm long and 110-120 cm wide. The surface of the blackboard should be smooth and non-glare. In primary grades, the blackboard is installed at a height of 85 cm from the floor, and in higher grades, at a height of 90 cm. The blackboard should be brown or dark green and have a shelf for chalk and a rag. A lamp is installed above the blackboard to provide good lighting. The teacher's desk and chair are placed in front of the first or middle desk.

classroom equipment is as follows:

1. Determine how much necessary and surplus equipment is in the classroom.

2. The quality and color of the parts are determined.

3. The quality and color of the board, as well as its height from the floor, are studied.

4. It is determined which group of desks or tables and chairs the children in the class will sit in.

5. Determine the distance between the rows of desks, the distance between the inner wall and the desk, the distance between the last desks and the wall, and the distance between the last desk and the board. The standard distance between the rows should be 70-75 cm., the distance between the inner wall and the desk should be 60 cm., and

the distance between the last desks and the wall should be 70 cm.

Control questions:

1. What is the height of the bottom edge of the blackboard from the floor in grades I-IV and in grades VX?
2. Explain the differences between tables and chairs manufactured according to the state standard (GOST) before 1971 and desks manufactured since 1975?
3. What should be the distance between the blackboard and the desks in the first row and between the desks in the last row and the blackboard? Explain the advantages and disadvantages?
4. What colors are appropriate for the desk?
5. What are the rules for sitting properly at a desk?

Tasks:

1. Table in the auditorium - chairs

Dimensions (cm):

Heigh t length	Desk cover height		Desk chair height		Slope position (degrees)	
	In practic e	Nor m	In practic e	Nor m	In practic e	Nor m

2. In the auditorium of equipment location

position (cm):

Blackboard						Desks					
Height		Color		1st grade and blackboa rd interval		Rows betwee n distanc e		Wall and desk interva l		Distanc e between the last desk and the wall	
In practice	Norm	In practice	Norm	In practice	Norm	In practice	Norm	In practice	Norm	In practice	Norm

3. Auditorium equipment :

No.	Equipment name	In the norm, necessary (+) or not necessary (-)
Auditorium No. _____, name ________________________________		
1		
2		
3		
4		
5		
6		

Hygienic assessment of lighting, heating and ventilation of educational institutions

Purpose of the work: to collect information on the lighting, heating, and ventilation of educational institutions and conduct a hygienic assessment based on standards.

Educational equipment: meter, centimeter tape, light measuring device (luxmeter), thermometer, data reflecting the norm.

Theoretical part: The floor area of the classroom should be 50 square meters. In grades 1-7, each room holds 40 students, and each student should have 1.25 square meters of floor space. In grades 8-9, each room holds 36 students, and each student should have 1.40 square meters of floor space.

The length of the classroom should not exceed 9 meters, otherwise students sitting at the last desk will have difficulty seeing the letters on the board. The width of the classroom should be 5.7-6.2 meters. If it is wider than this, less light will fall on the desks opposite the window. The height of the ceiling in the room should not be less than 3.5 meters, because the higher the ceiling of the classroom, the higher the windows can be built, which will make the classroom brighter.

Classroom lighting. As is known, classroom learning and writing activities are mainly related to manual labor. If the classroom lighting is good, eye fatigue does not occur quickly, and the student's working capacity increases. On the contrary, if the lighting is poor, the eyes get tired quickly, and the working capacity decreases. Doing exercises in a classroom with insufficient lighting for several months causes the student's eyesight to gradually deteriorate.

Classroom lighting is natural and artificial. Natural light is sunlight coming through windows. The natural light coefficient should be 1:4 or 1:5, meaning the total window area should be 12.5-10 square meters, which is a quarter or a fifth of the classroom floor area (50 square meters).

The height of the lower part of the window from the floor level should not exceed 80-85 cm. Light falls on the desks on the opposite side of the classroom from the window from the upper part of the window. Therefore, it is required that the upper part of the window be built closer to the ceiling, that is, only 20-30 cm lower than it. Classroom windows should be placed in such a way that the width of the wall gap between them does not exceed 30-50 cm, otherwise the desks in this place will receive little light.

Classroom lighting is determined using a special device. In addition, classroom lighting largely depends on whether the windows are built in accordance with hygienic requirements. To determine this, when standing on the opposite side of the classroom from the window and looking at the window, if its entire surface is easily visible, it is known that the window is built in accordance with the requirements, which means that the natural lighting of the classroom is assessed as good; if the sky is visible from 2/3 of the window, the classroom lighting is satisfactory, and if the sky is visible from only ½ or less of the window, the classroom lighting is assessed as unsatisfactory.

For artificial lighting of the classroom, spiral electric lamps or, in recent years, mainly fluorescent lamps are used. For every 1 m2 of floor space of the classroom, 36-48 watts of electric power should be provided. So, the floor space of the classroom is 50 m2, which should be illuminated by 6-8 spiral electric lamps with a power of 300 watts each. Electric lamps are placed in two rows on the ceiling. The distance between them should be the same. The height of the lamps from the floor should be 3 m. It is recommended to use fluorescent lamps for classroom lighting. When spiral electric lamps are used, the illumination of the classroom should be 150 lux, and when fluorescent lamps are used, 300 lux. In drawing rooms, 200 and 400 lux are required.

Classroom air and temperature regime. The carbon dioxide content of classroom air should not exceed 0.07-0.1% (normal air contains 0.03-0.04%). An increase in carbon dioxide in the air causes rapid fatigue of the nervous system of students and a decrease in learning. Especially in winter, some students in primary grades fall asleep during lessons. This is due to the increase in carbon dioxide in the air of the room.

During breaks and during lessons, the air in the classroom should be refreshed. For this, frames or louvres are installed on the windows. The total area of the louvre should be 50/1 of the floor area (if the floor area of the classroom is 50 m2, the area of the louvres on its windows should be 1 m2).

In a classroom, each student needs 4.5-5 m3 of air. During a one-hour lesson, 16-26 m3 of air is required per student. Therefore, in winter, during lessons, the air should be refreshed by opening the windows or transoms frequently (every 10-15 minutes for half a minute), and in the warm season, the classroom windows should be completely opened during lessons.

The temperature in the classroom should be 16-180 C, and the relative humidity should be 40-60%.

I. Hygienic assessment of natural and artificial lighting:

1. The light should fall on the pupils from the left.

2. The ratio of the glazed surface of the windows to the floor level is calculated. The standard light coefficient should be 1:4, 1:6.

3. The height of the window sill relative to the floor should normally be 80-85 cm, and the distance between the windows should be 50-75 cm.

4. The standard color of the ceiling, walls, doors, and frames should be white, the length of

the panel should be 1.30 cm, and the color should be light yellow, light airy colors.

5. To determine whether there is enough natural light in the darkest part of the classroom, have the student read a book there from a distance of 30-35 cm. If the student can read the book without difficulty, natural light is sufficient; if it is difficult, artificial lighting should be used.

6. The room may be illuminated with incandescent or fluorescent lamps. The power of the electric bulbs in the room should be 2100-2400 watts or 175-350 lux per 50 m2. The blackboard may be specially illuminated.

II. Hygienic assessment of classroom heating:

1. The rooms are heated by a special stove or central heating system.

2. Use a thermometer to measure the temperature of the room, hallway, wardrobe, and gym. The ideal classroom temperature should be -

17-19°C in winter, 23-24°C in spring, and 24-26°C in autumn, while the gym should be 15-16°C and have a humidity of 40-60%.

III. Hygienic assessment of natural and artificial ventilation:

1. The number and total size of windows in the room are calculated. The standard ratio of the floor area to the window area should be 1:50.

2. The standard width of the windows should be 0.6 m and the height should be 0.5 m.

3. After each lesson, students will learn how to ventilate the room using a fan.

4. There are special ventilation pipes that must be in working order.

5. Artificial ventilation or ventilation systems must be available in chemistry, physics, and biology laboratories and workshops.

Control questions:

1. What should the natural light coefficient be?

2. How many lux should the classroom lighting be when using spiral electric lamps or fluorescent lamps?

3. What percentage of carbon dioxide should not be contained in classroom air?

4. How much air is required for a student during a one-hour lesson?

Tasks:

1. Calculate the audience coverage and fill in the tables.

Natural lighting				Artificial lighting	
With Paul window window surface ratio	Window shelf height	Color of ceiling, walls, doors and frames	Panel length (cm.)	Incandescent lamp (watts or lux)	Fluorescent lamp (watts or lux)

In practice	Norm	In practice	Norm	In practice	Norm	In practice	Norm	In practice	Norm	In practice	Norm

2. Fill in the table based on the information about classroom heating.

Heating with a special stove or central heating system (+, -)		Classroom temperature						The temperature of the gym and humidity (^{0}C and %)	
		In winter (^{0}C)		In spring (^{0}C)		In autumn (^{0}C)			
In practice	Norm	In practice	Norm	In practice	Norm	In practice	Norm	In practice	Norm

3. Hygienicly assess the ventilation of classrooms and fill in the table.

The ratio of the floor surface to the window surface		Window size (cm.)		Ventilation by the Yelvizak method (+, -)		The presence of ventilation pipes (+, -)		Presence of artificial insemination or ventilations (+, -)	
In practice	Norm	In practice	Norm	In practice	Norm	In practice	Norm	In practice	Norm

Practical exercise 8. Hygiene of educational work. Hygienic assessment of the lesson and lesson schedule

Purpose of the work: To study the mental capabilities of students based on the hygiene of educational work, to determine the amount of normal educational workload.

Educational equipment: Class schedules for various classes, information reflecting the norm.

Theoretical part: The structure of the lesson and the organization of the school day are important for maintaining optimal mental performance. Its duration, difficulty, and boredom require a proper alternation of types of activities that require different activities from students.

Academic activities place significant demands on the body of schoolchildren. In this regard, the duration of classes should be appropriate to the age and capabilities of the children. At a young age, working capacity begins to decline 1.5 hours after the start of classes, and at middle and senior school age - after 2-3 hours, especially by the 6th lesson.

In this regard, the duration of lessons is an important factor in the hygienic organization of the educational process. According to physiologists and hygienists, a lesson for first-graders should not exceed 35 minutes, and for older classes - 45 minutes. According to psychologists, a 6-10-year-old child can concentrate for about 20 minutes, and a 10-12-year-old child for about 25 minutes. These studies confirm the need to organize lessons in such a way that the types of work alternate. For example, in a reading lesson, expressive reading should be replaced with question-and-answer, viewing didactic material, retelling, and in addition, since the first signal system is well developed in primary school students, it is possible to widely use exhibits and didactic teaching aids in the lesson.

The number of lessons is of great importance in the hygienic organization of school education. According to the current curriculum, 4 lessons per day are planned for grades 1-3, 4-5 for grades 4, and 5.6 lessons per day for grades 5-9.

To properly organize education, it is very important to distribute lessons throughout the day and week and to properly create a lesson schedule.

Depending on the ease and difficulty of mastering, all subjects are conditionally divided into very difficult, moderately difficult, and easy subjects.

The first very difficult subjects	*foreign language, mathematics*
For difficult secondary subjects	*physics, chemistry*
For secondary subjects	*history, natural science, native language and*

	literature, geography
Easy-to-learn subjects	*physical education, labor, singing, painting,* etc.

In the first hour of the school day, subjects of moderate difficulty should be taught, in the 2nd and 3rd hours the body's working capacity is at its highest, so it is recommended to teach subjects that are difficult to master during these hours. In the 4th hour, students show signs of fatigue. Therefore, teaching subjects that are easy to master (physical education, labor, singing, painting) in the 4th hour of the school day allows for a further increase in working capacity, and finally, if subjects of moderate difficulty (history, natural science, native language and literature, geography) are taught during the 5th and 6th hours, it will be better to master them.

Students' learning capacity also varies throughout the week. On the first day of school after a day off, the student's body is not yet fully mobilized for work. Therefore, difficult subjects should be avoided on the first day of school if possible. On the 2nd and 3rd days of school, the body's working capacity is at its highest, and it is better to do difficult subjects and tests on these days.

Starting from the 4th day of study, the body's working capacity begins to decrease, but on the 6th day of study, there is almost no decrease in performance. This means that if on the 4th day of study, light subjects related to movement are taught, and educational hours and excursions are held on this day, students will rest, as a result, their working capacity will be significantly restored on the 5th and 6th days of study, which will allow more difficult subjects to be included in the lesson schedule on the 5th and 6th days of study.

Measures to prevent fatigue during mental work during class:

1. The teacher explains new material at a time when the student has optimal working capacity;

2. In the second half of the lesson, using active teaching methods to explain without keeping the student's attention on one subject for a long time;

3. Constantly changing teaching methods;

4. Ventilate classrooms during breaks;

5. Involve students in various tasks and make extensive use of educational technology tools, strictly adhering to their rules;

6. Use of didactic teaching aids in explaining lesson material;

7. Conduct physical education classes between classes;

8. Organize the lesson with high pedagogical skills, explain in a cheerful mood, and speak in different tones.

The lesson schedule is an important part of the learning process. Properly compiling a lesson schedule prevents students from becoming mentally exhausted. The lesson schedule must meet several hygienic requirements, which are:

- set age-appropriate lesson times:

- putting subjects that require a lot of mental effort after subjects that require physical effort;

- on Monday, reduce the number of subjects that require a lot of mental effort;

- Avoiding subjects that require a lot of mental effort on Saturday.

Control questions:

1. What do you consider important in organizing school education in a hygienic way?

2. Into how many types are all subjects conventionally divided, depending on the ease and difficulty of mastering?

3. How many hours should the total weekly workload of classes be for children of primary school age?

4. What are some subjects that are easy to learn?

Tasks:

1. Fill in the table based on the information about the student's mental working ability periods.

Periods	Time (min .)	Signs	Teacher's activities
Start-up period			
Optimal working period			
Full, compensation period			
Unstable compensation period			
A period of progressive decline in activity			

2. Fill in the table based on the teacher's qualities.

No.	Teacher characteristics	Positive (+, -)	Negative (+,-)
1	Passing the lesson in high spirits	+	-
2			
3			
4			
5			
6			
7			
8			
9			
10			

2. Create a lesson schedule for ______ class (course) based on the hygienic requirements for the lesson schedule.

Monday	Tuesday	Wednesday

1. ________	1. ________	1. ________
2. ________	2. ________	2. ________
3. ________	3. ________	3. ________
4. ________	4. ________	4. ________
5. ________	5. ________	5. ________
6. ________	6. ________	6. ________

Thursday	Friday	Saturday
1. ________	1. ________	1. ________
2. ________	2. ________	2. ________
3. ________	3. ________	3. ________
4. ________	4. ________	4. ________
5. ________	5. ________	5. ________
6.	6.	6.

____________________ ____	____________________ ____	____________________ ____

Practical exercise 9. Hygienic assessment of the daily routine

Objective: To develop students' skills in creating a daily routine based on hygienic requirements for the routine.

Educational equipment: Information about the student's personal agenda, hygiene requirements for the agenda.

Theoretical part: When creating a daily routine for children and adolescents, it is necessary to take into account the alternation of work and rest, changes in the types of activities. Under the influence of favorable environmental conditions, the body of children and adolescents grows and matures. When the daily routine is properly organized, the child does not get tired. When the daily routine is followed, conditioned reflexes are formed in the nervous system, and children become disciplined and orderly. When the daily routine is not followed, the child experiences fatigue, insomnia, loss of appetite, nervous breakdowns, and a decrease in working capacity.

The daily routine for first and second shift students in general secondary schools is drawn up taking into account their age. This includes proper organization of rest, sleep, meals, extracurricular activities, assistance with household chores, school activities, etc.

Homework should be appropriate for the child's age. It is recommended that 1st graders be given 45 minutes of homework, 2nd graders 1-1.5 hours, 3rd and 4th grades 2-2.5 hours, and 5th-

10th grades 3-3.5 hours. When doing homework, it is necessary to take a break in the fresh air every 45 minutes. After returning from school, it is necessary to eat and play active games, and take a walk in the fresh air. Then homework can be prepared. After completing homework, students should help with homework. However, they should not be busy with homework and not do their homework or get tired. It is necessary to teach students from a young age to clean their beds, put their clothes in order, and take a bath in the evening and in the morning.

Sleep is an important part of the daily routine. The child should eat 2-2.5 hours before bedtime. After dinner, he should take a short walk in the fresh air. It is not recommended to do strenuous mental work, play exciting games, or watch TV before bedtime.

Lower-grade students can watch TV 3-4 times a week, 1-1.5 hours a day, and upper-grade students can watch it 4-5 times a week, 2-2.5 hours a day, sitting 2-2.5 m away from it, maintaining proper posture. It is not allowed to watch TV lying down or on your side. Elementary school students should go to bed between 8 and 9 o'clock, and students in grades V-VII between 9:30 and 10:00. The bed should be clean and not too soft. The room temperature should be 18-20 ° C, and in winter the window should be open. In the summer, children should sleep in the fresh air in the yard or on the veranda.

It is necessary to eat at a certain time every day, so that when the time for eating approaches, the appetite appears, and the food is digested quickly and well. If you do not eat on time, the appetite decreases. The food that a child eats in a day should cover the energy spent by his body.

Students approximate day order

Day order structural parts	1st – 4th grade (time)	5-7- class (time)	8th - 11th grade (time)
Morning from sleep stand	7. 00	7. 00	7. 00
Morning physical education , exercise treatments (wiping , showering) place collection , washing	7. Up to 30	7. Up to 30	7. Up to 30
Morning breakfast	7. Up to 50	7. Up to 50	7. Up to 50
To school road to take	8. Up to 20	8. Up to 20	8. Up to 20
At school lessons	8.30-12.30	8.30-14. 00	8.30-14.00
From school return or walk to do	Until 13.00	14.30 until	Up to 15
Lunch	13. 30	14. 30	15. 30
Holiday (7 years old) children for sleep (open) in the air walking , moving games	Until 14.30	15.00 until	Until 16.00
Home tasks preparation	Until 16.00	16.00 until	Until 17.00
Open airborne walks and games	17. 30 to	19.00 until	20. 00 until
Home tasks preparation	Until 19.00	20.00 until	Until 21.00

Evening food , free exercises (book) study , home to their work help to give , music hearing)	Until 20.00	Until 21.00	21. Until 30
To sleep preparation and the room ventilation	20. 30	21. 30	Until 22.00
Night sleep	21. 00	22. 00	22. 30

In some large schools, a special "health improvement class" is established for children with weakened health, where students from the same grade are grouped together and taught, and a special, simplified schedule is created for them.

Control questions:

1. What should be the daily routine of children with weakened health along with healthy children?

2. What can be achieved as a result of a daily routine based on hygiene requirements?

3. For whom is a special simplified agenda created?

4. What should a teacher pay attention to when giving homework to a child?

Tasks :

1. Create a schedule for upperclassmen.

No.	Activity type	Time interval
1	Awakening	
2	Physical education	
3	Breakfast	
4	School lesson	
5	Big break. Lunch.	
6	Second lunch	
7	Housework (free physical activity)	
8	Homework	
9	Dinner	
10	Cultural leisure	
11	Homework	
12	Evening walk	
13	Slccp	

2. Provide a scientific justification for your daily routine. ____________________ _

_

____

______________________ ______

____

______________________ ______

____

_______________________ _______

3. Write your schedule on a calendar.

No.	**Activity type**	**Time interval**
1		
2		
3		
4		
5		
6		
7		
8		
9		
10		
11		
12		
13		
15		
16		
17		
18		

4. Explain whether your daily routine is structured correctly or incorrectly: _______________

Determining the type of higher nervous activity

The purpose of the work: to determine the temperament of students through the G.Yu. Eysenck test and develop skills for an individual approach to them.

Educational equipment: G.Yu. Eysenck test, information about higher nervous activity - temperaments.

Theoretical part: *Sanguine:* Will laugh out loud at inconsequential things. An unimportant fact will cause him severe anger. Responds with a quick and strong excitement. Quickly concentrates his attention. Highly active, very energetic and hardworking, can work for a long time without getting tired, enthusiastically takes on new tasks. It is easy to call him to discipline. He can quickly control his emotions and involuntary movements. He is quick-witted, quickly takes on new tasks. His mind works quickly, is resourceful. His feelings, moods, interests and aspirations are very changeable. He easily adapts to new conditions. He can quickly move from one task to another. He has an extroverted nature.

Choleric: Uncontrollable, impatient,

restless, irritable, and impulsive. Sharp and demanding in dealing with people. Able to solve problems, not always working at the same pace, risk-taker. Has great determination, has difficulty focusing. Fast-paced. If he starts something, he will finish it, but if he is interested in it, he will not.

Phlegmatic: Has low emotional excitability, is difficult to make laugh, anger, or upset. Does not break his calm even when a major unpleasant event occurs. Has few gestures, is characterized by energy, hard work, endurance, perseverance, and self-control. His activity, pace of movements, and speech are slow and expressionless. He concentrates his attention slowly. He shifts his attention with difficulty. He adapts to new conditions with difficulty. Introvert.

Melancholic: Tears flow from his eyes for no apparent reason. He is extremely irritable and cries slowly. Sincere, laughs very little, is inactive. He is not confident, shy, and if there is a slight difficulty, he will wash his hands and scold himself. He is not enthusiastic, not determined. His attention is easily distracted, he is unstable. His mental tempo is slow. He has an introverted nature.

G. Yu. Eysenck's test for determining temperaments

You will be offered a test consisting of 57 questions. You must answer these questions only with "Yes" or "No". There are no "good" or "bad" questions. Therefore, try to answer without thinking too much. To make the answering process faster and easier, you can put a "+" plus sign for the "Yes" answer and a "–" minus sign for the "No" answer.

1. Do you often have a tendency to experience new impressions?

2. Do you often feel the need for friends

who understand you and encourage you when you need it?

3. Are you a free person?

4. You have a hard time saying "no" to others. Is that true?

5. Do you think for a long time before doing something?

6. When you promise to do something, do you always keep your promise, regardless of whether it is convenient or inconvenient for you?

7. Do you often have mood swings or highs?

8. Usually you without thinking some the work as or some the word saying Will you send it ?

9. Sometimes you no how without reason yourself in the world unhappy from people You think it 's one . Is that right ?

10. You in dispute swallowed exit for no from something You won't return . Is that right ?

11. You have beautiful , handsome with a man (woman) to talk correct if you want , you can do it yourself somehow discomfort feeling Do you notice ?

12. You sometimes yourself manage unobtainable at the level you are angry exit cases become Is it worth it ?

13. You have one momentary mood under the influence behavior done increase cases become Is it worth it ?

14. You have often this the work not to do need was or this the word not speaking need was , - said worry cases become Is it worth it ?

15. People with talking from sitting according to book to read acceptable You'll see . Shy, right ?

16. You sad to do Is it easy ?

17. You various to be in circles (in companies) Do you like it ?

18. You have from others wants to hide was

thought , ideas become Is it worth it ?

19. You have sometimes to work was strong passion suddenly laziness status with exchange cases become Is it worth it ?

20. You are in a narrow circle only to yourself good familiar was your friends to be acceptable Do you see ?

21. Do you often daydream?

22. If someone yells at you, do you immediately respond?

23. Do you often feel guilty?

24. Are all your habits good and pleasant?

25. Do you have thc ability to be relaxed and have fun in circles?

26. Do you consider yourself an impressionable and emotional person?

27. Do others always consider you to be cheerful and cheerful?

28. After you accomplish something

important, do you ever feel a nagging feeling that you could have done it better?

29. Do you tend to be quiet around other people?

30. Do you sometimes gossip?

31. Do you sometimes have trouble sleeping because of all the thoughts that come to your mind?

32. If you want to know something, it's easier for you to read about it in a book than to ask people, right?

33. Do you have frequent heart palpitations even when you are not physically active?

34. Do you enjoy tasks that require you to sit for long periods of time and concentrate your attention and thoughts?

35. Do you have tremors in your hands and feet due to excitement?

36. Would you pay for the transportation of your luggage if you knew for sure that there was

no inspector?

37. Do you like being in circles where you joke around with each other?

38. Are you short-tempered?

39. Do you like doing things that require you to be fast-paced?

40. Do you ever have any anxiety because of thinking about unpleasant events that may happen in the future?

41. Do you usually walk slowly and leisurely?

42. Have you ever been late for work or a meeting?

43. Do you often have nightmares?

44. They say that you love talking to people so much that you try not to miss the opportunity to talk to strangers. Is that true?

45. Do you suffer from any physical pain?

46. Would you consider yourself unlucky if you were deprived of the opportunity to talk to other

people?

47. Do you consider yourself a nervous person?

48. Is there anyone you know that you clearly dislike?

49. Can you look at yourself as a confident person?

50. Do you get upset easily when people point out your personal or professional shortcomings?

51. Do you believe that you cannot get true satisfaction from attending various parties?

52. Do you often feel uncomfortable with the feeling, "I'm not like everyone else?"

53. Do you have the ability to breathe life into a boring routine?

54. Do you sometimes talk about things you don't understand?

55. Do you worry about your health?

56. Do you like to play jokes on others?

57. Do you ever suffer from insomnia?

Results analysis

1. The scale determining the level of reliability of the answers:

"Yes" - 6, 24, 36. "No" - 12, 18, 30, 42, 48, 54.

2. Extraversion-introversion scale:

"Yes" - 1,3,8,10,13,17,22,25,27,39,44,46,49, 53,56.

"No" - 5,15,20,29,32,34,37,41,51.

3. Emotional stability scale:

"Yes"- 2,4,7,9,11,14,16,19,21,23,26,28,31,33,35,38,40,43,45,47,50,52.55, 57 .

If the answers obtained on the scale determining the level of reliability of the answers are higher than 5 points, then it is considered that the person taking the test did not answer from the heart, and the accuracy of the results is not guaranteed.

The answers that match this key are then calculated and reflected in the table below.

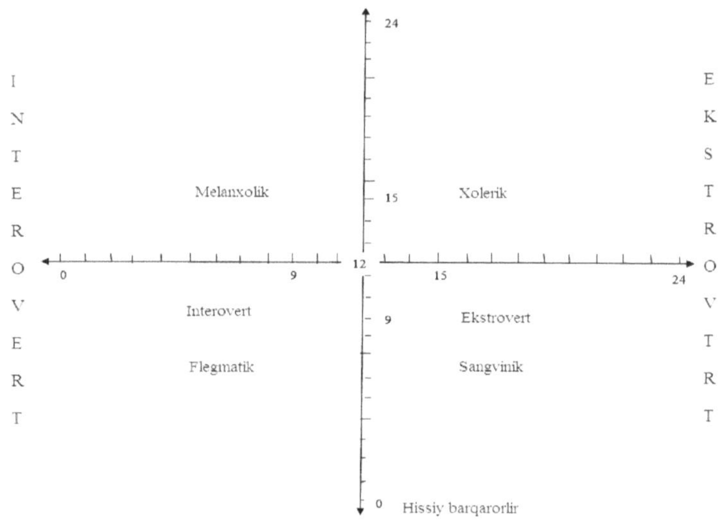

Tasks :

1. G.Yu. Eysenck in the test to questions given answers based on the table fill in ("Yes" +, " No " –)

Que stion	1	2	3	4	5	6	7	8	9	10	11	12	13	14	15

number															
Answer sign (+, –)															
Question number	16	17	18	19	20	21	22	23	24	25	26	27	28	29	30
Answer sign (+, –)															
Question number	31	32	33	34	35	36	37	38	39	40	41	42	43	44	45
Answer sign (+, –)															
Question number	46	47	48	49	50	51	52	53	54	55	56	57			
Answer sign (+, –)															

2. Determine the level of confidence based on the question numbers shown below.

The scale determining the level of reliability of the answers:

"Yes" - 6, 24, 36. "No" - 12, 18, 30, 42, 48, 54. (If the answers are higher than 5 points, the correctness of the results is not guaranteed).

3. Below shown question numbers based on points count (each number 1 point) .

" Yes " - 1,3,8,10,13,17,22,25,27,39,44,46,49,53,56

" No "-5,15,20,29,32,34,37,41,51.

Emotional-stability scale :

"Yes"- 2,4,7,9,11,14,16,19,21,23,26,28,31,33,35,38,40,43,45,47,50,52,55,57.

Harvest was numbers based on graphic :

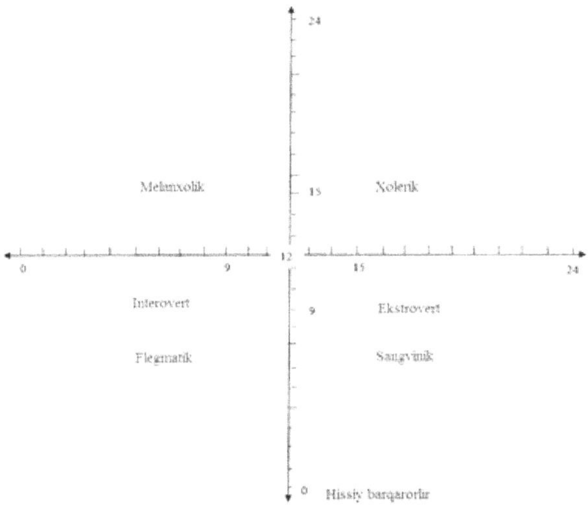

References

1. Aripova S.H. “Physiology and hygiene of youth”. T.: “Science and technology”. 2010.
2. Ismailov MN “Hygiene of children and adolescents”. T.: “National Encyclopedia of Uzbekistan” State Scientific Publishing House. 1994.
3. Makhmudov E. “Adolescent Physiology and School Hygiene”. T.: Teacher. 1994.
4. Sodiqov K., Aripova SX, Shakhmurova GA “Physiology and hygiene of youth”. T.: Yangi asr avlodi. 2009.
5. Adolf Faller ., Michael Sch u enke -The Human Body - “ An Introduction to Structure and Function” ThiemeStuttgart· New York http: // www.bestmedbook.com/ 2004

Table of Contents

www.ingramcontent.com/pod-product-compliance
Lightning Source LLC
Chambersburg PA
CBHW062143160726
48282CB00027B/925
* 9 7 8 9 3 6 9 0 8 1 0 3 5 *